Y

I wanted to show my

so I've put together a free gift for you.

The 'Your Body is Your Gym' Bonus Pack

Just visit the link below to download it now.

www.GoodLivingPublishing.com/bodyweight

I know you will love this gift.

Thanks!

Peter Paulson

Contents

Introduction 9

Why Bodyweight Training? 12

    Workout Anywhere & Anytime...12

    Get the Abs You Always Wanted 13

    Stop the Injury Cycle 14

    Build Lean, Hard Muscle While Burning Fat 15

    Save Money..16

Building The Body You Want..17

    Steps to Ensure Your Success..17

Your Guide to Nutrition 19

    Excerpt from The 6 Pack Chef 20

    Example Recipes 25

        Bacon Avocado Omelette 25

        Scallop & Vegetable Kabobs 27

        Shrimp Stir Fry..28

        Garlic Baked Tilapia..29

Program Overview 30

    Week by Week Program Overview 35

The Movements 38

Abdominal & Core Exercises 39

    Plank..40

    Side Plank 41

    Crunches 42

    Arms Extended Crunch 43

    Leg Raises..44

    Toe Touchers...45

    Side Jack-knife...46

Ab Hold 47

Back Exercises 48

Under Table Row 49

Back Extension 50

Superman 51

Bicep Exercises 52

Bicep Towel Curls 53

Chest Exercises 54

Push Up 55

Incline Push Up 56

Push Up with Twist 57

Diamond Push Up 59

Side to Side Push Up 60

Spiderman Push Up 62

Forearm Exercises 63

Towel Twist 64

Leg Exercises 65

Air Squat 66

Reverse Lunge 67

Glute Bridge 69

Single Leg Glute Bridge 70

Calf Raises 71

Jump Squats 72

Jumping Lunges 73

Pistol Squat 74

Shoulder Exercises 75

Pike Push Up 76

Shoulder Rotations 77

Hindu Press Up...78

Wall Shoulder Press 80

Tricep Exercises...81

Wall Press...82

Advanced Wall Tricep Press 83

Explosive Tricep Press 84

Cardio...85

Mountain Climbers 86

High Knees 87

Burpees 88

Skipping...89

Star Jumps 90

The 8 Week Routines Program 91

Beginner..92

Week 1 92

Session 1..93

Session 2..94

Session 3..95

Session 4..96

Week 2 97

Session 1..98

Session 2..99

Session 3..100

Session 4..101

Week 3 102

Session 1..103

Session 2..104

Session 3..105

Session 4..106

Week 4 107

Session 1..108

Session 2..109

Session 3..110

Session 4..111

Week 5 112

Session 1..113

Session 2..114

Session 3..115

Session 4..116

Week 6 117

Session 1..118

Session 2..119

Session 3..120

Session 4..121

Week 7 122

Session 1..123

Session 2..124

Session 3..125

Session 4..126

Week 8 127

Session 1..128

Session 2..129

Session 3..130

Session 4..131

Intermediate & Advanced.............................132

Week 1 132

Session 1...133

Session 2...134

Session 3...135

Session 4...136

Week 2 137

Session 1...138

Session 2...139

Session 3...140

Session 4...141

Week 3 142

Session 1...143

Session 2...144

Session 3...145

Session 4...146

Week 4 147

Session 1...148

Session 2...149

Session 3...150

Session 4...151

Week 5 152

Session 1...153

Session 2...154

Session 3...155

Session 4...156

Week 6 157

Session 1...158

Session 2...159

Session 3...160

Session 4..161

Week 7 162

Session 1..163

Session 2..164

Session 3..165

Session 4..166

Week 8 167

Session 1..168

Session 2..169

Session 3..170

Session 4..171

Introduction

Hi,

I just want to say thank you for buying my book, I've worked long and hard on this in order to make it of absolutely phenomenal value to you and I can't wait to go on this journey with you.

Before we dive into the book and get started I want to take a few moments to just mention one or two quick points.

Clients, friends and family members often ask me if fitness is really "all that important" and after I fight the urge to give them a reality check in the form of a slap I calmly explain the following…

Your health and fitness is arguably the most important aspect of your life. By living a healthy life you are basically wearing a Kevlar vest towards the majority of life's bullets. Not only does it protect you from physiological dangers such as heart disease and diabetes, but it also protects you psychological health. Regular exercise and a healthy diet have been shown to reduce stress, reduce anger and reduce tensions, but that's not all, it's also shown to improve your sleep quality and your massively increase your happiness in life.

So, yes, health and fitness really is "all that important."

What a healthy lifestyle looks like to each individual person differs massively but for the majority of us it means eating well most of the time and exercising regularly.

We all have our own reasons for wanting to be in better shape and be healthier, and whatever your reasons are I applaud you. The simple act of picking up this book shows you're more dedicated towards your health, life and wellbeing than the vast majority of people.

But as you have picked up this book I want to let you know what to expect by reading and implementing the advice presented.

In this book I will be covering the following topics:

- The benefits of bodyweight training and why it's an excellent choice

- How to build the body you want

- Nutritional and dietary advice, plus sample recipes

- An 8 week body re-composition plan to get you in your best shape ever

- 40 images of the exercises you need to perform during the 8 week plan

And much, much more.

If you go through this book and implement what I suggest then I guarantee that you will see incredible results. The leading reason for people not succeeding in reaching their health and fitness goals is they slack off - don't be that person. Follow the 8 week program and stick to it, each week is designed for a specific reason and ignoring them will lead to poorer results.

To date I've written three #1 bestselling books and my rationale for this book is that I feel it's something the market needs.

I wanted to focus on a book about bodyweight training as it removes any barriers that people may have towards working out – cost of a gym membership, lack of time etc.- it is my hope that this book will encourage more people to exercise, and ultimately live a better life.

Don't get me wrong, gyms are great and I would never say otherwise but I know they're not for everyone and I particular love bodyweight training for a number of reasons that will be discussed later.

Anyway, I think I have talked long enough, so it's time to dive into the book and change your body, life and health.

Enjoy.

Your friend,

Peter Paulson

Why Bodyweight Training?

You might be wondering why bodyweight training is so good or why anyone would consider it when they could just join a gym. Well, I want to take this chapter to address why bodyweight training is so incredible and how it can change your life.

I want to mention that I don't have any issues with gyms, in fact, I love working out in a gym, but I also love having the flexibility to work out anywhere. Whether it's at home, work, whilst travelling, or out in the local park. The flexibility to exercise efficiently and effective anywhere is incredibly freeing.

But now I want to just note down some of the reasons you are going to love bodyweight training and dive into them a little deeper.

Workout Anywhere & Anytime

Given that bodyweight training simply uses your body, you can literally workout anywhere you are, with no equipment. This is incredibly freeing as you are no longer tied down to your gym's location.

I know you live a busy a life and sometimes you just don't have the time to travel to the gym, get in a workout, and make it home in the time you have available. With bodyweight training this is never an issue again – all you need is a small amount of floor space. Plus, there is no need to factor in an extra 30 minutes for commuting back and forth. And if you still want to work out at your gym, well as you're taking your body to the gym, you can do bodyweight training there, and what's awesome is that you'll never need to wait on a machine to free up again.

Once you adopt bodyweight training you will start to notice that you almost never miss a workout. This is due to the fact that you've removed multiple psychological barriers for not exercising. You've also removed the common excuses people tout for not being able to work out. You will never hear yourself say, "It's too wet outside to go to the gym," "The gym is always too busy at this time," or "I've only got 30 minutes to spare, I can't get to the gym and workout in this time." Nope, with bodyweight training you've completely eliminated these excuses and you will find yourself never missing a workout.

Get the Abs You Always Wanted

When you go through a bodyweight training regime like this one, you will see your abs appear faster than you thought possible. Bodyweight routines are highly metabolic in nature and also engage your core in almost every exercise. This means that as you go through the routine you are consistently strengthening your core whilst shredding fat from your belly.

Combine these two factors with an excellent eating plan (coming up soon) and you will be showing off your new 6 pack quicker than you would have imagined.

Stop the Injury Cycle

Nowadays it seems like having an injury is in vogue, and I'm not talking about a serious injury such as torn rotator cuff, I mean those small twinges and pains people get in their knees, shoulders and elbows.

I'm sure you know what I mean and if you don't, just carry out a little observation next time you're at the gym. Watch somebody doing the chest press, after they rack the weight watch them as the rotate their shoulder and stretch it out with a grimace on their faces.

These little injuries are so incredibly common it's ridiculous and they all stem from one of the following: trying to lift too much weight, poor form and under developed stabilizing muscles from overusing machines.

Bodyweight training helps to solve all these problems.

You won't be attempting to lift stupidly heavy weights that are purely to stroke your ego. Instead you will be using strategically designed lifting time frames to work the muscles just as hard as if you had loaded the barbell with plate after plate.

As bodyweight exercises incorporate a huge number of your stabilizer muscles, you will be strengthening these every workout and preventing future injury, as well as building muscle.

The above points merge into the fact that with bodyweight routines you will not be lifting under poor form. Most people give up good form in their attempts to continually stack plates onto the bar. With bodyweight training you won't have the opportunity to do this. Throw in the continued development of your stabilizer muscles and you will always be exercising under excellent form.

There is a common misconception that in order to build muscle and lose fat you must have a gym membership, along with this goes the fact that you must take every supplement under the sun. Well, guess what... this is just marketing doing what it does best, convincing you of something in order to extract money from you.

The truth is, yes gyms are good and yes supplements are good, but you need neither.

In order to get in truly phenomenal shape you only need to do the following:

Break your muscles down and then rebuild them with proper nutrition.

That's it. You don't need a fancy piece of equipment or supplements X,Y, and Z.

By properly utilizing your bodyweight you will be placing your body in the correct environment to prime it for muscle growth. And as you work through this program you will be doing very specific things in order to place your body in the correct environment.

As I mentioned earlier, bodyweight training is highly metabolic, but that's not the only way you will be losing fat. As this program will be helping you build muscle you will also lose fat as a direct result of having more muscle. Increasing the amount of lean muscle on your body will increase your metabolism and testosterone levels – both of which are proven to decrease the amount of fat your carry.

Save Money

If you're working out at home, the office, or your local park, one thing is going to remain constant –you will be saving money. No spending money on gas to get to the gym, no pricey gym memberships, no extortionate personal trainers.

Again, I'm not saying you have to quit your gym, but if money is tight and you still want to get in brilliant shape, then feel free to quit the gym and pocket that extra $50 per month.

Building The Body You Want

Each of us have specific goals and body re-composition targets we want to hit. We all have that image in our head of how we want our bodies to look. We've seen the celebrity we want to look like and we have set some sort of rough date that we want to achieve it by.

Having these visions and goals is crucially important to your success in any new fitness regime. If you don't have the end goal in sight you won't have the motivation and drive to reach the finish line.

Before you start this program, I want you to answer some very simple questions and write the answers to them down. Doing this will help to clarify your goals and set them in stone. Understanding your motivations is one of the most important steps you can take in order to reach the successful conclusion of any goal.

So, before you get started on the program work your way through the following steps.

Steps to Ensure Your Success

- Write one specific sentence describing exactly how you want your body to look.

Is it lose 10lbs? Add 3 lbs of muscle? Tighten your stomach? Drop to single digit body fat %? Your goals are personal to you so don't let anyone else influence your decision, just write down what you personally want.

- Find an image of the body you want to achieve and print it out, keep it somewhere you will see it every day.

Doing this is a powerful visualization exercise and will help keep you motivated as you can now physically see your end goal.

- Take a picture of your body.

Throughout the program you are going to look at this image so you can see just how far you've came. Having an image of your body before you start the program means you will have proof of progress and this will help to further motivate you throughout the journey.

- Ask yourself why you are wanting to change your body and write the reasons down.

Doing this helps you understand the rationale behind your desire to change and this is what you can focus upon if you ever want to quit. If you ever have a day you want to give up then go back and read this statement.

By going through each of these quick steps you have drastically increased your chances of success. By clarifying and visualizing your goals you will find that you are much more motivated than you've ever previously been. Now that you have the end result in sight you just need an excellent program to follow and that's what this book is going to provide for you.

Your Guide to Nutrition

Losing fat, building muscle, and crafting the body of your dreams can't be done with just an exercise and fitness routine. Your diet and nutrition is just as important as the exercise you do.

Without a solid nutritional plan you will never get the body you want. I cannot emphasize the importance of proper nutrition in regards to health and fitness.

Not only will it allow you to reach your body composition goals, but it will also make you happier, help you sleep better, increase your testosterone, and improve almost every health marker we measure. Perhaps, more important than all those combined, is that it will help you live longer; simply put, people who eat a healthy diet live longer.

In this program you will see results if you only follow the exercises, but in order to see incredible, life changing results I suggest you follow the principles I am going to lay out.

The following section is lifted from my #1 bestselling book, The 6 Pack Chef." The focus of this book was nutritional rules and recipes for rapidly cutting body fat to reveal your 6 pack. I have lifted out the nutritional rules from this book as they are the exact rules I suggest you follow whilst going through this program. I've also provided a few example recipes, if you want to see the full collection of recipes you can purchase, The 6 Pack Chef at Amazon.com. Additionally, as part of your free gift you also receive five more '6 pack' recipes, check out the front of the book for more details.

Nutritional Rules to Follow

This section will explore the various rules you have to follow in order to shred off fat and reveal your 6 pack. These rules are simple to follow and you will most likely have come across some of them before.

Read them carefully and follow them religiously.

The first few rules are all set around the famous (and very true) saying of, "Abs are made in the kitchen, not the gym."

The key to getting truly shredded is through the correct approach to diet. So without further ado, here are your nutritional rules.

You Have to Eat.

If you want to be lean and have a shredded 6 pack you have to eat. Starving yourself will just result in a loss of muscle, a screwed up metabolism and a malnourished appearance. By eating you will be providing your body will everything it needs to burn fat, keep your metabolism working, feed your muscles, and ultimately get shredded – but remember you need to eat the right foods, which brings us to rule 2.

Eat the Right Foods

Unless you are a freak of nature or on steroids you won't be able to get shredded by eating whatever you like. You need to base your diet around whole foods and avoiding manufactured/processed foods. (Check out your free gift for a shopping list of foods.)

Whole foods can be considered anything that isn't packed full of additives and came out of a factory. Sure the packet of cooked chicken at the grocery store might boast 30g of protein, but look closer at the nutritional info and you will see a long list of additives – these will prevent you ever getting truly lean.

Conversely, eating natural whole foods (nuts, grass-fed beef, organic chicken, eggs, beans, legumes etc.) will give your body the nutrients it requires to burn the stubborn fat hiding your abs.

Going 100% natural can be very difficult and is not essential, instead you should aim for 80% whole-foods. This means you can still eat (in small doses) things like hot sauces, certain breads etc. This 80/20 split will help you stick to your diet, not go crazy, prevent cravings and save you money.

Every Meal Must Have a Protein Source

Being shredded is not just about losing body fat, you also need to have a substantial amount of muscle. Lean muscle burns fat, the more muscle you have the more fat you burn and the building block of muscle is protein.

When you are on the quest to reveal your abs you will be in a calorie deficit (expending more calories than you take in) and when in a deficit protein will carry out the following functions:

- Keep you feeling fuller longer as protein aids satiety and prevents hunger.

- Prevent muscle breakdown from calorie reduction.

Eat Greens & Keep Fibre High

The fibre you get from green vegetables and carbs, such as legumes, have some excellent health benefits which make them essential for getting shredded. Eating more fibre has been proven to help you control weight fluctuations, lose weight quicker, promote a healthier heart, and increase your levels of satiety after a meal. Aim to eat some greens and fibre in every meal. As you go through the recipes in this book, you will notice how many of them call for these ingredients.

Don't Be Afraid of Fat

It seems counter intuitive, but eating fat helps you lose fat. Your body requires fat to function, it's a crucial building block, and ensuring you consume dietary fat will help you reach your goals faster. The main foods you want to derive your fats from are things like extra-virgin olive oil, steak, beef, chicken thighs, and avocado.

If you limit your fat intake too steeply then your body will go into "survival mode" and not let go of its existing fat stores as it is concerned no more is coming. Avoid this by accepting healthy dietary fats as an essential part of your diet.

Resistance Training

If you want to reveal your abs, you need to place your muscles under tension. As mentioned in the previous rule muscle burns fat, but there are other reasons you need to lift if you want to reveal your 6 pack:

- Resistance training is highly metabolic and torches fat.

- Increases testosterone – higher T levels are directly linked to an increase in fat burning.

- To build muscle, strength the core and increase the size of abdominal muscles.

Train Fasted (if possible)

If your schedule allows for it train early in the morning in a fasted state. Fasted state training has a plethora of benefits which will allow you to carve out your abs at an accelerated pace. The benefits of training early in the morning are shown below:

- Your testosterone levels are at their highest in the morning.

- You prime your body to burn fat for the remainder of the day.

- Any food you eat after working out will go straight to your muscles and not have the opportunity to turn to fat.

The benefits of training fasted will now be listed:

- Increase in production of HGH (human growth hormone).

- Your body targets fat cells for energy as no food is available for fuel.

- You will NOT have an insulin spike.

The first few times you train fasted will feel unusual, but by the 3rd or 4th session you will notice an increase in energy levels and performance in the gym. I recommended a large black coffee or double espresso (no sugar, cream etc.) before the gym to help with your energy levels.

Ensure you eat as soon as possible after your workout.

Refuel Every 7-10 Days

In order to strip away body fat and reveal your abs, it is essential that you are in a caloric deficit the majority of the time. However, it is also crucial that you 'refuel' every so often. A refuel day consists of greatly spiking your caloric intake in order to achieve the following:

- Reset your leptin levels.

- Boosts your metabolism.

- Replenish your glycogen stores.

Stop you losing your mind when cutting.

A refuel day is very important to anyone wanting to reveal their abs, but several things should be noted about the day. Do not confuse it with a 'cheat day,' you will still be eating the same healthy foods, just in greater amounts. Do not eat for the sake of eating, just eat more each meal. If you need to eat something sweet for the sake of your sanity, be very careful with the portion control.

Plan your refuel days ahead of time, decide what you are going to eat ahead of time and make sure you enjoy the feeling of the increase protein, carbs, and fats pulsing through your body.

Example Recipes

The full collection recipes can be found within, The 6 Pack Chef. Go to Amazon and search for, The 6 Pack Chef by Peter Paulson and you can check out the full book there.

Bacon Avocado Omelette

Ingredients

3 eggs, whisked

3 rashers of bacon

1 avocado, stone removed, skinned and chopped into chunks. You will only be using half.

½ red onion, finely chopped

Cilantro, finely chopped, around 1 teaspoon worth

Hot sauce, to taste

Directions

Cook bacon under the grill/broiler or in a pan.

As bacon cooks take your avocado chunks and add to a bowl. Mash the avocado slightly with a fork.

Add the onion and cilantro to the bowl and mix well.

Once bacon is cooked, cut it up and throw it in the bowl as well. Mix again.

In a greased pan over a medium heat add the eggs and leave to cook for 2 minutes.

Once the omelette begins to form and the middle isn't runny anymore. Scoop the avocado mixture onto one half of the omelette.

Fold the empty half over the avocado mix to complete the omelette.

Cook until ready.

Ingredients

5 oz. scallops, enough for 2-4 skewers

1 tablespoons extra-virgin olive oil

Juice from half of a lemon

½ teaspoon thyme

2 shallots, peeled and halved

2 bell peppers, cut into chunks

6 cherry tomatoes

½ zucchini, cut into rounds

Ground black pepper, to taste

Sea salt, to taste

Skewers, soaked in water

Directions

In a bowl combine the oil, lemon juice, thyme, salt, and pepper. Mix well and then add the scallops to this mixture and coat well. Leave to sit in this marinade for 20 minutes.

Whilst you marinade the scallops preheat your broiler/grill.

Skewer the vegetables and scallops in an alternating fashion.

Season with salt and pepper.

Place under grill and cook for about 2-3 minutes per side.

Shrimp Stir Fry

Ingredients

2 teaspoons garlic, minced or finely chopped

½ teaspoon ginger, ground or minced

3 Spring onions, chopped

Pak choi, torn

1 cup of king prawns, raw

1 bag of bean sprouts

2 tablespoons soy sauce

Half of a lemon, juiced

Sesame seeds

1 tablespoon extra-virgin olive oil

Directions

Place a wok over a medium heat and add the oil.

Once oil is heated, add the garlic, onion, and ginger. Cook for 2 minutes, stirring continually.

Throw the prawns in the pan and cook for 30 seconds, stirring continually.

Add the pak choi and bean sprouts and cook for 1 minute. Stirring frequently.

Once the prawns turn pink (a sign they are almost done) add the soy sauce, lemon juice, and a generous amount of sesame seeds.

Toss well and cook until the prawns are cooked fully.

Ingredients

2 tilapia, fillets

2 cloves garlic, crushed or finely chopped

3 tablespoon extra-virgin olive oil

1 onion, finely chopped

1 tablespoon cayenne pepper

Salt and Pepper, to taste

Directions

Lay the fish fillets in an oven proof dish. Rub them well with the crushed garlic.

Drizzle with the olive oil until well coated. Evenly lay the onion across the fillets.

Cover and refrigerate overnight or at least 6 hours.

Preheat oven to 350F.

Remove fish from oven. Sprinkle with cayenne, salt ,and pepper. Let fish come to room temperature, about 30 minutes.

Bake for 30 minutes

Program Overview

By now you're probably wondering what is the exact bodyweight program you're going to be following? Well, I've very briefly mentioned earlier what the program will focus on, but I am now going to dive a little deeper into it so that you know what to expect.

This program is specifically designed around using only your bodyweight to help you reach your goals.

It is laid out initially as an 8 week program, after that time you will have made significant gains and if you've followed the program progression and nutritional structure to a tee you will see incredible results. After the initial 8 weeks you can do a number of things: you can continue with the program, skipping the first several weeks, you can design your own bodyweight routines or you can adopt any new practice you like.

I've designed this program using a number of very specific strategies in order to accelerate your results by properly utilizing your body weight. Throughout the course of the program you will be using strategies such as progressive overload, reduction of rest times, lactic acid training, and muscle time under tension. Using these strategies in combination with highly metabolic routines that focus on multi-muscle movements will result in spectacular results.

In the paragraph above I mentioned the concepts of progressive overload, lactic acid training, and time under tensions (TUT), I will now elaborate further as to what these are, why they're so powerful and how they will help you reach your goals.

What is Progressive Overload?

Progressive overload is the very simple concept of continually increasing the demands you place upon your body in order to stimulate muscle growth. If you do not continue to increase the work done by your muscles then they will cease to grow.

If you want to increase muscle size and definition you must continue to break down your muscles by forcing them to do more work than previously done. Doing this causes your muscles to adapt and grow, if you choose not to increase the loads your muscles are undergoing then your muscle has no reason to grow.

Now the problem with most bodyweight programs is that increasing the load usually relates to increasing the weight you are using, and as your bodyweight is not going to massively increase these programs deliver poor results.

This program is completely different as it delivers progressive overload without the use of dumbbells, weight machines or barbells. The reason this program can do this by utilizing two specific types of training – time under tension and lactic acid training.

What is Time Under Tension Training?

Time under tension or TUT is a very specific type of training that was popularized by Tim Ferriss in his book, The 4 Hour Body. I won't go deeply into the details and science behind how TUT works and will instead just give a brief overview so that you can understand the concept and how it is going to help you.

TUT training relates to placing your muscles under stress for a specific amount of time in order to break them down. The lifting and lowering phases in TUT are tightly controlled and executed slowly and steadily, this differs from conventional lifting which generally places the focus on moving as much weight as possible through the desired motion, with no regards to lifting cadences.

But what are the benefits of TUT training?

Well, first off by having your muscles be under tension for an extended period of time the result will be a greatly enhanced metabolic response and an increase in the release of growth hormone.

Secondly, by strategically increasing the time muscles are under tension you will be more effectively depleting your muscles glycogen (stored carbohydrates) levels. This means that during your post-workout feeding window your muscles will be craving food, especially carbohydrates, in order to repair themselves and they will rapidly absorb it into your muscles – this means you can greatly increase muscle growth potential.

The above point also helps link to the next point which is fat loss. As TUT training places a great strain on muscle fibres it is highly metabolic, this means you will remain in a metabolic state for a massively increased length of time after your workout. This means that even when you're not working out you are still burning off fat.

With this bodyweight program you will be able to progressively overload your muscles without the need for gym equipment, instead you will simply use time.

Strategically increasing the stress your muscles are undergoing means that you can continue to promote growth by continually overloading your muscles and breaking down the fibres. This is one of the keys which will skyrocket your results over any other previous bodyweight program you've tried. No other bodyweight program utilizes strategies like TUT training and therefore gains plateau and results are poor.

Add in the final strategy you're going to be using at different stages in this program and you have the cocktail for growth and this final strategy is lactic acid training.

What is Lactic Acid Training?

In order to promote further progressive overload, fat loss, and incredible results you will also be using lactic acid training. This is a style of exercise that was popularized by the personal trainer and fitness model John 'Roman' Romaniello.

Again, like with TUT training, I won't go into the science behind lactic acid training and will instead give an overview providing you with exactly what you need to know.

Lactic acid training is incredibly powerful when it comes to promoting fat loss without the loss of muscle and without the hindrance of preventing muscle growth. The concept of this training is to promote higher production levels of lactic acid within your muscles. If you're not sure what lactic acid is then just think of that burning feeling you get deep in your muscles after a few tough reps, that's lactic acid, and we're going to be ramping up the production of that. This style of training isn't easy, but it is very beneficial.

So, how does lactic acid training work?

The 'burn' you've felt before is a result of your body using glycogen as an energy source. As glycogen breaks down it becomes a variety of different compounds and these compounds are the source of the 'burn' and they create lactic acid in your muscles.

As the levels of lactic acid increases, so too does your body's release of growth hormone. This is the perfect environment for muscle gain and fat loss as growth hormone causes fat cells to turn to fuel and causes muscles to grow.

So when your body is producing more lactic acid, it is placing you in the correct environment for muscle growth and fat loss; throw in a solid diet plan and you will see results faster than you believed possible.

Bringing it all Together…

As mentioned above, when you bring all these aspects together into a strategically designed program the results you will be able to see are great. Each stage of the program is designed so that your body is continually adapting, growing and changing.

In this next section I will give the structure of the program so you can see a week-by-week guide as to what you will be undergoing.

Week by Week Program Overview

This outline will give you a more detailed overview to the bodyweight program I've designed for you. Each week builds upon the previous, getting tougher and introducing new strategies. This ensures that you are continually progressing and forcing your body to adapt, build muscle, and shred fat.

Within each week of the program the weekly introduction will give further details on the strategies you will be using, it will also provide rep ranges, rest times, tension times, lifting cadences, and much more.

Each week has 4 exercise sessions and how you split these is up to you, however, I would recommend the following structure over the course of 7 days.

- Workout Day

- Workout Day

- Rest Day

- Workout Day

- Rest Day

- Workout Day

- Rest Day

I would not suggest working more than this as resting is incredibly important for body re-composition, it seems counterintuitive, but in order to grow and lose fat you need to stop working and allow the body to repair itself.

The Week by Week Structure

There is an option for either a beginner or intermediate/advance program. Choose the one which is best suited to your body type and current fitness levels. If you've never worked out before, or haven't in years, then do not attempt the intermediate/advance program – you will fail. The programs are very similar with key alterations having been made within each week to best suit the target group.

Weeks 1-2

The first phase of the program is focused upon priming your body for the next 6 weeks of intensity. Each workout is designed to prime your muscles for the strategies you will be using in subsequent weeks.

Weeks 3-4

In this phase we will be introducing time under tension training to the equation, you will now understand the intensity that comes along with constant muscle tension and see why you never need a gym again. Each week will reduce rest times and increase tension times to ensure progressive overload.

Weeks 5-6

In this phase we will be introducing lactic acid training to the equation. Lactic acid training will shock your muscles as you will never have experienced anything like this before. During this phase you will be ramping up your fat loss potential due to the production of mass amounts of lactic acid and the metabolic nature of the workouts.

Week 7

A return to time under tension training. Week 7 will be a direct repeat of week 4 in terms of exercises performed but the difference will come from the rest times and lifting times.

Week 8

A return to lactic acid training. Week 8 will be a direct repeat of week 6 in terms of exercises performed but the difference will come from the rest times and lifting times.

The Movements

Abdominal & Core Exercises

Plank

Main Muscle Targeted: Abdominals

How to Perform:

Get into the position shown below and hold for the specified amount of time. Tense your abdominals and continue to breathe normally, do not hold your breath. Do not arch your back, keep a straight line from your heels to shoulders.

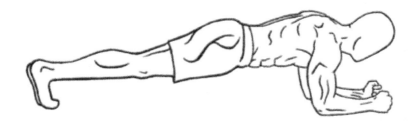

Side Plank

Main Muscle Targeted: Obliques

How to Perform:

Get in the position shown below and hold for the specified amount of time. Tense your core and continue to breathe normally, do not hold your breath. Do not prop your hips either up or down, keep a straight line from your heels to shoulder.

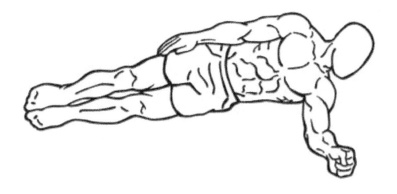

Crunches

Main Muscle Targeted: Abdominals

How to Perform:

Get into the position shown below. Contract your abdominals whilst raising your back off the floor, once your elbows meet your legs slowly lower yourself down and repeat. Aim to keep continually tension in the abdominals throughout the movement, release the tension briefly as your back returns to the floor.

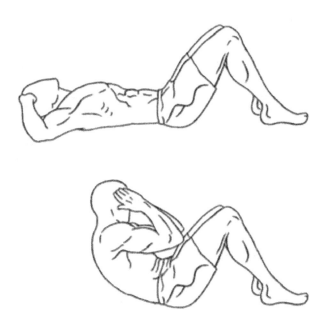

Arms Extended Crunch

Main Muscle Targeted: Abdominals

How to Perform:

Get in the position shown below. Contract your abdominals whilst raising your back off the floor, when only your lower back is touching the ground begin to lower yourself back down. Aim to keep continually tension in the abdominals throughout the movement, release the tension briefly as your back returns to the floor.

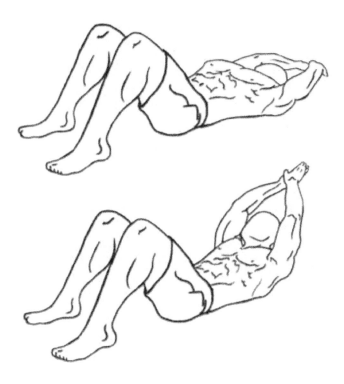

Leg Raises

Main Muscle Targeted: Abdominals

How to Perform:

Get in the position shown below. Keeping your upper body still begin to lift your legs off the ground. Once your legs reach the position shown below begin to lower them in a controlled fashion, do not just drop your legs. Do not let your heels touch the ground but instead stop them once 1" from the surface before lifting up again.

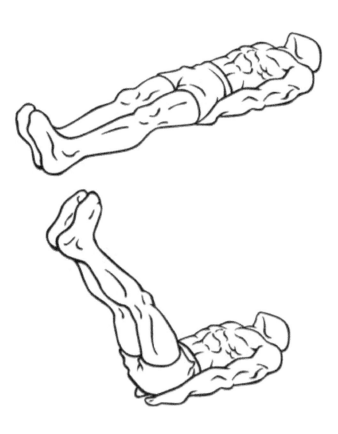

Toe Touchers

Main Muscle Targeted: Abdominals

How to Perform:

Get into the position shown below. Keeping your legs as still as possible in their current position reach upwards with your hands and try to touch your toes. Initially you may find it easier to lay your palms on your shins and then perform the move.

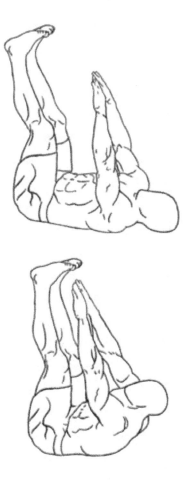

Side Jack-knife

Main Muscle Targeted: Obliques

How to Perform:

Get into the position shown below. Use the elbow that is touching the ground as a support to steady yourself and then simultaneously lift your leg upwards whilst moving your elbow towards it. If possible hold at the top of the movement for 1 second in order to increase the tension on your obliques.

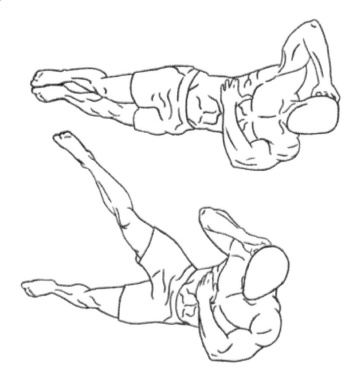

Ab Hold

Main Muscle Targeted: Abdominals

How to Perform:

Get into the position below. Breathe deeply outwards to expel air from your lunges and then without breathing in, pull your stomach upwards. Pull your stomach in tightly, as if you're trying to make your waist as thin as possible and hold for 1-2 seconds. Release and then repeat.

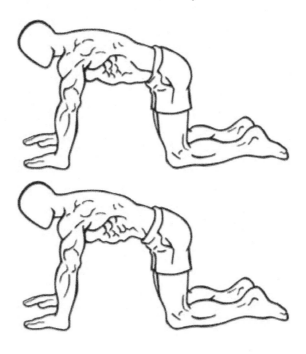

Back Exercises

Under Table Row

Main Muscle Targeted: Back

Secondary Muscles: Biceps, Forearms, Shoulders

How to Perform:

Get into the position as shown below but instead of gripping a bar grip the edge of a sturdy table. You should now be lying on the ground with your legs extended under your table. Keeping your heels pressed firmly against the ground start to pull your chest up towards the table. Once you reach the position shown in the second image lower yourself down until your back touches the ground.

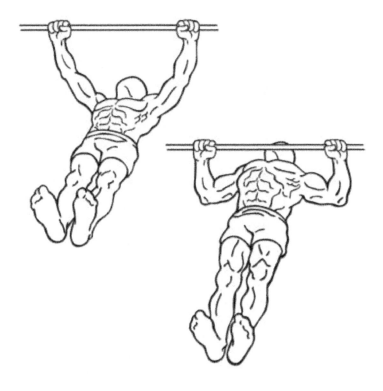

Back Extension

Main Muscle Targeted: Lower Back

Secondary Muscles: Abdominals

How to Perform:

Get into the position shown below. Whilst keeping your palms on the floor and lower body in position, pull your shoulders back to slightly arch your back.

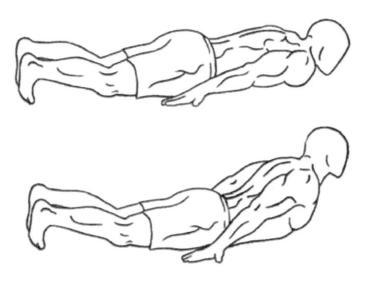

Superman

Main Muscle Targeted: Lower Back

Secondary Muscles: Abdominals

How to Perform:

Lie in the position shown below. Simultaneously pull your shoulders back and your legs up so that you're back and legs make a slight bow shape as shown below.

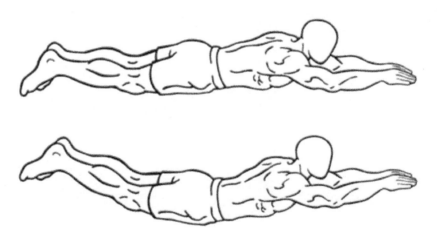

Bicep Exercises

Bicep Towel Curls

Main Muscle Targeted: Biceps

Secondary Muscles: Forearms

How to Perform:

Hold each end of a towel as shown below in the first image. You might want to spin the towel into a tight roll before doing this to avoid chance of it ripping. Place your foot at the middle point of the towel. Start to pull upwards on each end of the towel whilst applying downward force with your foot. The amount of pressure you apply with your feet is the amount of force your biceps will need to overcome. Switch feet every few repetitions.

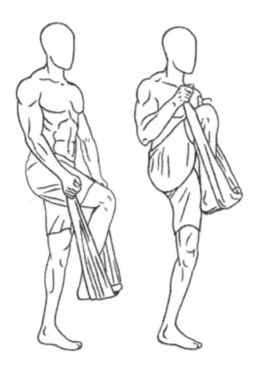

Chest Exercises

Push Up

Main Muscle Targeted: Chest

Secondary Muscles: Shoulders, Triceps

How to Perform:

Get into the position shown below. Hands should be spread slightly wider than your shoulder breadth. The line from your heels to shoulders should be straight, and should remain straight throughout the movement, to achieve this and stop your back arching keep your core tight. Lower your chest towards the ground in a controlled manner until your upper and lower arms form a 90° angle. Push your body back up to the starting position.

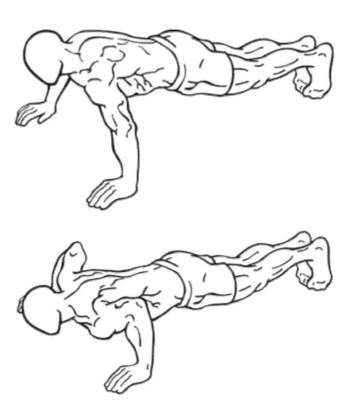

Incline Push Up

Main Muscle Targeted: Chest

Secondary Muscle: Shoulders, Triceps

How to Perform:

Get into the position shown below. Hands should be spread slightly wider than your shoulder breadth. The line from your heels to shoulders should be straight, and should remain straight throughout the movement, to achieve this and stop your back arching keep your core tight. Lower your chest towards the ground in a controlled manner until your chest is a few inches from the ground. Push your body back up to the starting position.

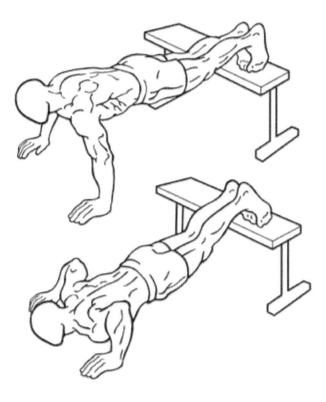

Push Up with Twist

Main Muscle Targeted: Chest

Secondary Muscle: Shoulders, Triceps, Abdominals, Obliques

How to Perform:

Complete the push up movement as described in previous push up exercises except at the top of the movement when you will further tighten your core and rotate one arm off the ground until body is in position shown in image 3. With each push up alternate the arm you rotate upwards to ensure you work both sides equally.

Image is shown on next page.

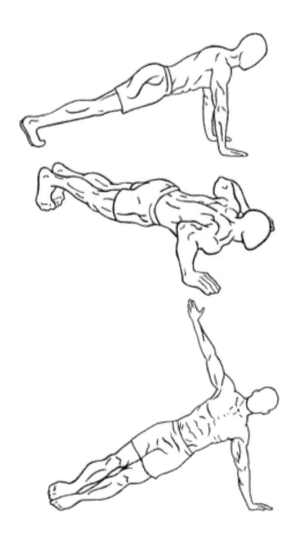

Diamond Push Up

Main Muscle Targeted: Chest, Triceps

Secondary Muscles: Shoulders, Abdominals

How to Perform:

Get into the position shown below. Hands should be in a rough diamond shape. The line from your heels to shoulders should be straight, and should remain straight throughout the movement, to achieve this and stop your back arching keep your core tight. Lower your chest towards the ground in a controlled manner until your upper arms are parallel to your torso. Push your body back up to the starting position.

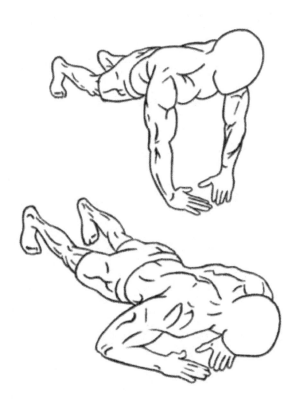

Side to Side Push Up

Main Muscle Targeted: Chest

Secondary Muscles: Shoulders, Triceps

How to Perform:

Get into the position shown below. Hands should be spread slightly wider than your shoulder breadth. The line from your heels to shoulders should be straight, and should remain straight throughout the movement, to achieve this and stop your back arching keep your core tight. Lower your chest towards the ground in a controlled manner, as you lower yourself start to lean to one side and put the majority of weight on one arm and one pectoral muscle. Once you reach the position shown in image two, push back up to the starting position. Alternate sides with each repetition.

Image shown on next page:

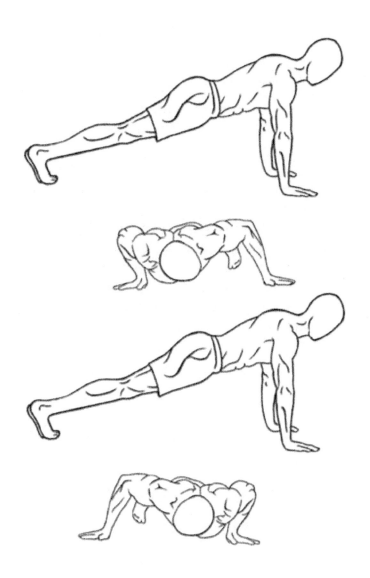

Spiderman Push Up

Main Muscle Targeted: Chest

Secondary Muscles: Abdominals, Shoulders, Triceps

How to Perform:

Get into the position shown below. Hands should be spread slightly wider than your shoulder breadth. The line from your heels to shoulders should be straight, and should remain straight throughout the movement, to achieve this and stop your back arching keep your core tight. Lower your chest towards the ground in a controlled manner whilst simultaneously bring one knee up to meet your elbow. As you push back towards the starting position return your foot to the floor. Alternate each side for each repetition.

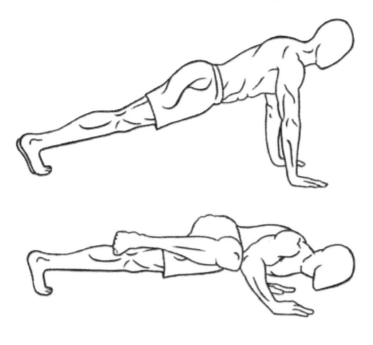

Forearm Exercises

Towel Twist

Main Muscle Targeted: Forearms

How to Perform:

Wrap a towel into a roll and grip it tightly in each hand. Twist your hands in opposite directions to engage your forearms. Twist and hold before releasing the tension in your forearms, repeat.

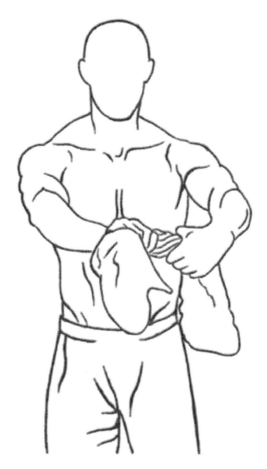

Leg Exercises

Air Squat

Main Muscles Targeted: Legs - *Quadriceps, Gluteus, Hamstrings*

Secondary Muscles: Calves, Abdominals

How to Perform:

Stand with feet slightly wider than shoulder width apart and toes pointing slightly out. Lower yourself down whilst raising your arms forward until your achieve the position shown in the second image. Upper legs should be parallel to the floor before you drive yourself back upwards to the starting position. Keep your core engaged throughout the movement to stabilize yourself.

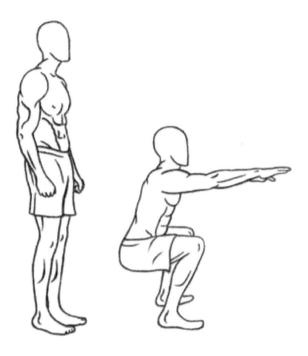

Reverse Lunge

Main Muscles Targeted: Legs –*Quadriceps, Gluteus, Hamstrings*

Secondary Muscles: Calves, Abdominals

How to Perform:

Stand with feet shoulder width apart. Extend one leg backwards whilst lowering yourself until you are in the position shown in the second image. To return to starting position drive upwards with the majority of the force coming from your leading leg (the one not extended backwards). Keep your core engaged throughout the movement to stabilize yourself. If you can't keep your arms by your side during the movement try extending them outwards to provide balance.

Image is shown on the next page:

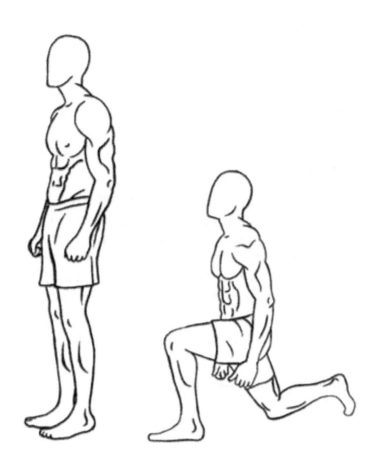

Glute Bridge

Main Muscle Targeted: Gluteus

How to Perform:

Lie down in the position shown below. Drive your butt upwards whilst keeping upper body and lower legs still. Tense your butt at the top of the movement and then lower in a controlled fashion to the starting position.

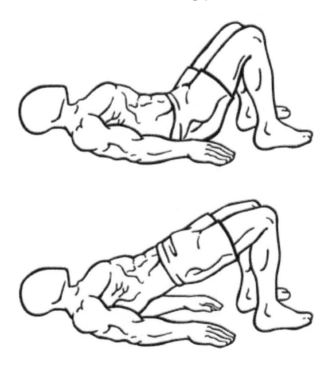

Single Leg Glute Bridge

Main Muscle Targeted: Gluteus

How to Perform:

Lie down in the position shown below. Drive your butt upwards whilst keeping upper body and lower legs still. Tense your butt at the top of the movement and then lower in a controlled fashion to the starting position. Alternate legs for each repetition.

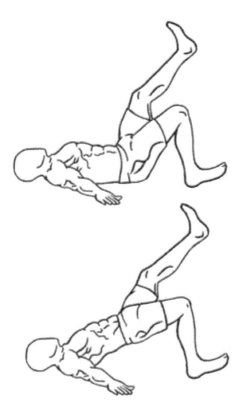

Calf Raises

Main Muscle Targeted: Calves

How to Perform:

Stand with feet shoulder width apart. Push off the ground the base balls of your feet until your heels are extended off the floor. Lower yourself back into position. You may initially need to place your hands against a wall for support when doing this move.

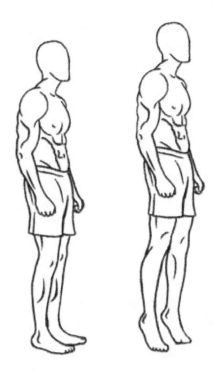

Jump Squats

Main Muscles Targeted: Legs - *Quadriceps, Gluteus, Hamstrings*

Secondary Muscles: Calves, Abdominals

How to Perform:

Stand with feet slightly wider than shoulder width apart and toes pointing slightly out. Lower yourself down into the squat position and then explode upwards so that you're feet come completely off the ground by several inches. Land on the balls of your feet and lower yourself back into the squat position in a controlled fashion. Repeat.

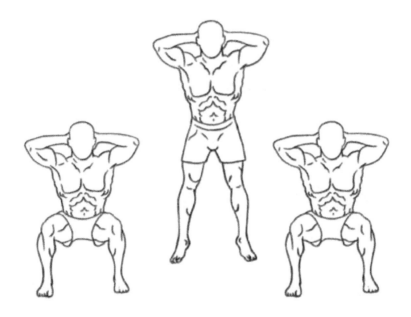

Main Muscles Targeted: Legs – *Quadriceps, Hamstrings, Gluteus*

Secondary Muscles: Calves, Abdominals

How to Perform:

Perform a reverse lunge as previously explained in "Reverse Lunge" up until the point you are about to return to the starting position. Instead of standing up, explode upwards so that you're fully off the ground. Whilst in the air switch your legs so that your foot that was previously extended backwards is now extended forward.

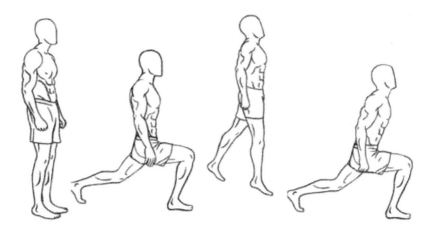

Pistol Squat

Main Muscles Targeted: Legs - *Quadriceps, Gluteus, Hamstrings*

Secondary Muscles: Calves, Abdominals

How to Perform:

Note: This is a very advanced move. If you can't do it then revert back to an air squat.

Stand with feet slightly wider than shoulder breadth. Raise one leg off the ground as shown in the first image and carefully bend forward until you're in the position shown in the second image. From this position lower yourself into the completed position. Drive upwards from this point and swing your arms backwards to help propel yourself up. Switch legs and repeat.

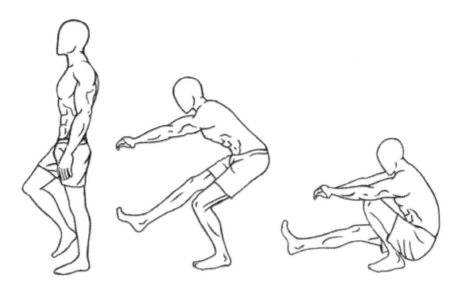

Shoulder Exercises

Pike Push Up

Main Muscle Targeted: Shoulders

Secondary Muscles: Triceps

How to Perform:

Get into the position shown below. Hands should be slightly wider than your shoulder breadth. Carefully lower your face towards the ground with the tension being kept in your shoulders. Push upwards with your arms to return to the starting position.

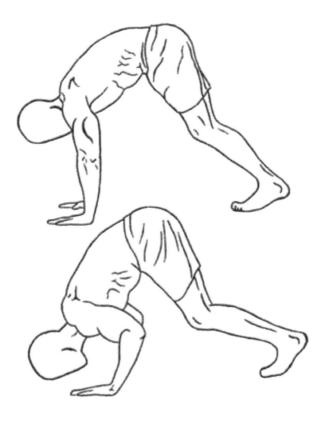

Main Muscle Targeted: Shoulders

How to Perform:

Extend arms outwards and make small rotations for the pre-specified amount of time.

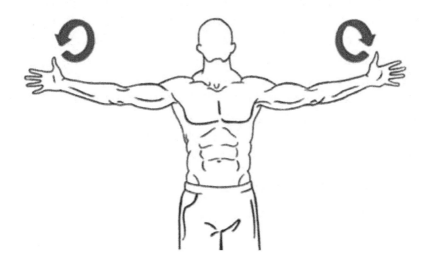

Hindu Press Up

Main Muscles Targeted: Shoulders

Secondary Muscles: Chest, Triceps, Abdominals

How to Perform:

Get into the position as shown in the first image. Allow your body to move forward, in a controlled fashion, until you are in the position shown in the second image. At this point begin to arch your back upwards so that your arms are locked out at the top of the movement. Go through the following movements in reverse to return to the starting position. *Although it is hard to describe in writing this movement should be completed in a single flowing movement. If you need further advice I would suggest searching Youtube for a video.*

Image shown on the next page:

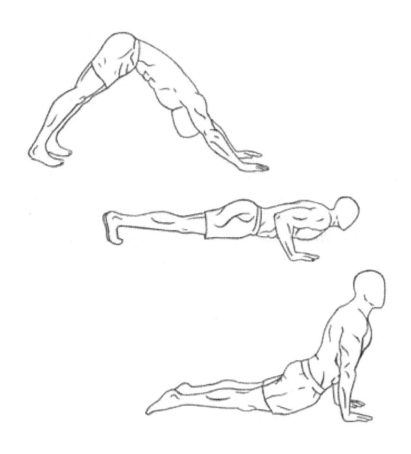

Wall Shoulder Press

Main Muscles Targeted: Shoulders

Secondary Muscles: Triceps

How to Perform:

Place your hands slightly wider than shoulder width apart. Begin to walk your feet up the wall until your arms are fully extended. Do not aim to go completely vertical. Once you are in position lower your head towards the ground and then drive upwards with your arms to return to the starting position.

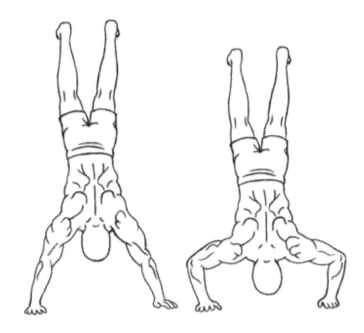

Tricep Exercises

Wall Press

Main Muscle Targeted: Triceps

How to Perform:

Place your hands against the wall in a diamond shape. Walk your feet backwards until you are in the position shown in the first image. Extend your arms, engaging your triceps until your arms are fully extended. Return to the initial position and repeat.

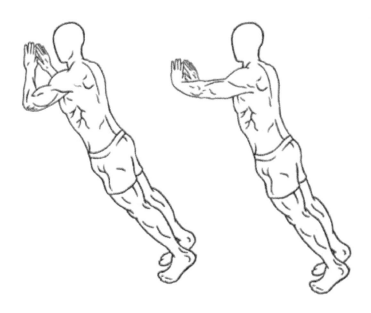

Main Muscle Targeted: Triceps

Secondary Muscles: Shoulders

How to Perform:

Get into the same position as the regular tricep press, except this time aim to walk your legs back much further. Repeat the same plane of motion as the regular tricep press but aim to go much deeper, so that your forearms are resting flat against the wall, your head should be in between your forearms and close to the wall. Drive your arms forward against the wall to return to the starting position.

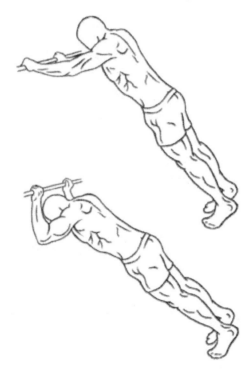

Explosive Tricep Press

Main Muscle Targeted: Triceps

How to Perform:

Get into the position shown in the first image. The line from your heels to shoulders should be straight, and kept straight throughout the whole movement, achieve this by engaging your core. When ready to perform the move place your palms flat on the ground and explosively push upwards so that you end up in the second position. Lower yourself back to the starting position in a controlled fashion.

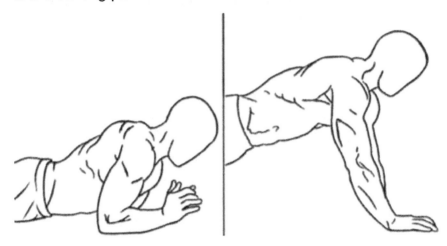

Cardio

Mountain Climbers

How to Perform:

Get into the position shown below. Keep the line from your heels to shoulders straight. Draw one knee at a time up to the position shown below in the second image then return to the starting position. Repeat this with your other leg and then continue to repeat in a rapid fashion.

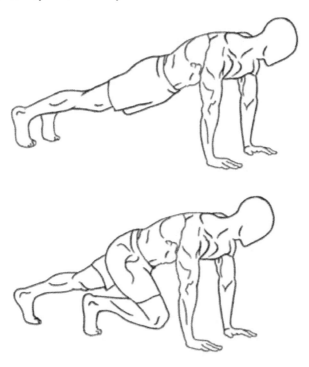

High Knees

How to Perform:

To perform this move imagine yourself running on the spot but aim to bring your knees as high as possible. Repeat on the spot for as long as the time specifies.

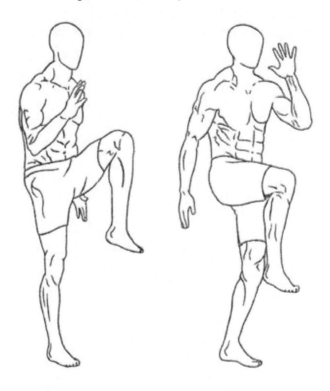

Burpees

How to Perform:

From the starting position squat into the position shown in the second image. From here drive your legs backwards rapidly until you are in position three. Explosively pull your legs back into position four and then explosively drive upwards into an air jump. Return to the starting position and repeat.

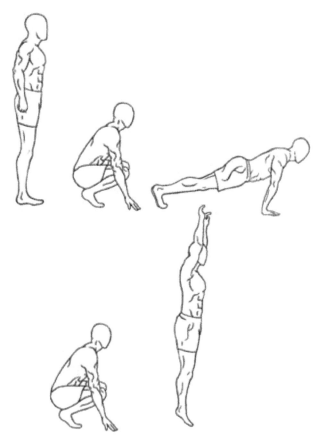

Skipping

You can perform this with or without skipping ropes.

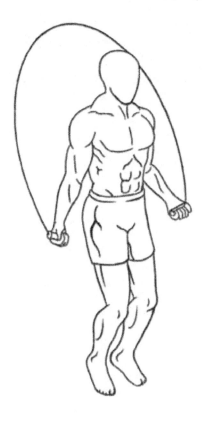

Star Jumps

How to Perform:

From a standing position explosively jump upwards and extend your arms and legs so your body makes a star shape. Before you land draw your arms and legs back into the starting position and land carefully. Repeat.

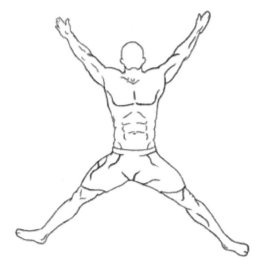

The 8 Week Routines Program

Complete each exercise in the order listed below.

Aim for the target repetitions (reps) specified and depending on fitness level rest 0-30 seconds between exercises.
Repeat the circuit for the specified number, i.e. "*Circuit 1: x4*" means that you will repeat this circuit 4 times before moving onto the next circuit.

After completing the full circuit rest 30-60 seconds before repeating.

Wait 60-90 seconds between moving from one circuit to the next.

Circuit 1: x3

Air Squats	7-10 reps
Pike Push-ups	5-8 reps
Plank	15 secs
Glute Bridge	8 reps
Air Squats	5-8 reps

Circuit 2: x3

Push-ups	7 reps
Reverse Lunges	5-8 reps
Calf Raises	15-20 reps
Shoulder Rotations	30 secs
Plank	15 secs
Air Squats	5 reps

Circuit 3: x3

Pike Push-ups	5-8 reps
Shoulder Rotation	20 secs
Tricep Wall Press	10-15 reps
Air Squats	5-10 reps

Circuit 1: x3

Reverse Lunges	7-10 reps
Leg Raises	5-10 reps
Under Table Row	5-8 reps
Towel Bicep Curl	8-10 reps
Glute Bridge	7 reps

Circuit 2: x3

Under Table Row	5-8 reps
Plank	20 secs
Push-ups	7-10 reps
Back Extension	5-8 reps
Towel Twist	10 reps

Circuit 3: x2

Air Squats	8-10 reps
Shoulder Rotations	30 secs
Towel Bicep Curl	10 reps
Superman	5-8 reps

Session 3

Circuit 1: x3

Air Squats	7-10 reps
Push-ups	8-10 reps
Plank	20 secs
Tricep Wall Press	10-15 reps
Towel Bicep Curl	8-10 reps

Circuit 2: x3

Reverse Lunges	5-8 reps
Pike Push-ups	5-8 reps
Tricep Wall Press	10-15 reps
Leg Raises	5-10 reps

Circuit 3: x3

Push- ups	7-10 reps
Superman	5-8 reps

Circuit 1: x2

High Knees	10-20 reps
Mountain Climbers	10-20 reps
Leg Raises	5-8 reps
Crunches	8-10 reps
Plank	30 secs
Skipping	30 secs

Complete each exercise in the order listed below.

Aim for the target repetitions (reps) specified and depending on fitness level rest 0-30 seconds between exercises.
Repeat the circuit for the specified number, i.e. "*Circuit 1: x4*" means that you will repeat this circuit 4 times before moving onto the next circuit.

After completing the full circuit rest 30-40 seconds before repeating.

Wait 60-70 seconds between moving from one circuit to the next.

Circuit 1: x4

Air Squats	8-10 reps
Pike Push-ups	6-8 reps
Plank	25 secs
Glute Bridge	10 reps
Lunges	8 reps

Circuit 2: x3

Push-ups	8-10 reps
Reverse Lunges	8-10 reps
Calf Raises	20 reps
Shoulder Rotations	45 secs
Plank	20 secs
Air Squats	7-10 reps

Circuit 3: x3

Pike Push-ups	8 -10reps
Shoulder Rotation	30 secs
Tricep Wall Press	15 reps
Air Squats	8-10 reps

Session 2

Circuit 1: x3

Reverse Lunges	10 reps
Leg Raises	8-12 reps
Under Table Row	8 reps
Towel Bicep Curl	8-10 reps
Single Leg Glute	7 reps

Circuit 2: x3

Under Table Row	6-8 reps
Plank	30 secs
Push-ups	8-12 reps
Back Extension	8 reps
Towel Twist	12 reps

Circuit 3: x2

Air Squats	10 reps
Shoulder Rotations	45 secs
Towel Bicep Curl	12-15 reps
Superman	6-8 reps

Circuit 1: x3

Air Squats	10 reps
Push-ups	10-12 reps
Plank	30 secs
Tricep Wall Press	15 reps
Towel Bicep Curl	10-15 reps

Circuit 2: x3

Reverse Lunges	5-8 reps
Pike Push-ups	5-8 reps
Tricep Wall Press	10-15 reps
Leg Raises	5-10 reps

Circuit 3: x3

Push-ups	10 reps
Superman	8 reps
Side Plank	15 secs

Circuit 1: x3

High Knees	10-20 reps
Mountain Climbers	10-20 reps
Leg Raises	5-8 reps
Crunches	8-10 reps
Plank	30 secs
Skipping	30 secs

Circuit 2:

Burpees	Until failure

Complete each exercise in the order listed below.

Aim for the target repetitions (reps) specified and depending on fitness level rest 30-45 seconds between exercises. Repeat the circuit for the specified number, i.e. *"Circuit 1: x4"* means that you will repeat this circuit 4 times before moving onto the next circuit.

Where you see "TUT", this stands for time under tension and states the length of time for a given exercise. So, TUT 5x3 would mean 5 seconds for the first part of the exercise followed by 3 seconds for the second part i.e.:

"Air Squats – TUT 5x3" would result in a 5 second lowering phase, followed by 3 seconds lifting to return to starting position.

For TUT movements aim to complete at the very least 2 repetitions but ideally 4.

After completing the full circuit rest 60 seconds before repeating.

Wait 90 seconds between moving from one circuit to the next.

Circuit 1: x3

Air Squats	TUT 3x3
Pike Push-ups	TUT 3x3
Reverse Lunges	TUT 3x3
Single Leg Glute	TUT 3x3
Plank	30 secs

Circuit 2: x3

Jumping Lunges	5 reps
Hindu Push-ups	5 reps
Calf Raises & Hold	8 reps
Shoulder Rotations	45 secs
Side Plank	30 secs
Reverse Lunges	5 reps

Circuit 3: x2

Diamond Push-ups	5-7 reps
Ab Hold	5 reps
Air Squats	5-8reps

Circuit 1: x3

Under Table Row	TUT 3x3
Reverse Lunges	8-10 reps
Leg Raises & Hold	5-8 reps
Towel Bicep Curl	TUT 3x3
Single Leg Glute	5-8 reps

Circuit 2: x3

Under Table Row	TUT 3x3
Side Plank	30 secs
Push-ups	8-10 reps
Back Extension	5 reps
Towel Twist	10-12 reps
Shoulder Rotations	45 secs

Circuit 3: x2

Pike Push-ups	10 reps
Towel Bicep Curl	10-12 reps
Air Squats	5-8 reps

Circuit 1: x3

Push-ups	TUT 3x3
Plank	30 secs
Jump Squats	5 reps
Tricep Wall Press	TUT 3x3
Reverse Lunges	5 reps

Circuit 2: x3

Lunges	7-10 reps
Pike Push-ups	TUT 3x3
Diamond Push-ups	3-5 reps
Leg Raises	8-10 reps

Circuit 3: x3

Incline Push-ups	5-8 reps
Superman	5 reps
Glute Bridge & Hold	10 reps

Circuit 1: x3
No rest between exercises

Mountain Climbers	20 reps
Leg Raises	10 reps
Mountain Climbers	15 reps
Crunches	8 reps
Mountain Climbers	10 reps
Side Jack Knife	5 reps

Complete each exercise in the order listed below.

Aim for the target repetitions (reps) specified and depending on fitness level rest 30-45 seconds between exercises. Repeat the circuit for the specified number, i.e. *"Circuit 1: x4"* means that you will repeat this circuit 4 times before moving onto the next circuit.

Where you see "TUT", this stands for time under tension and states the length of time for a given exercise. So, TUT 5x3 would mean 5 seconds for the first part of the exercise followed by 3 seconds for the second part i.e.:

"Air Squats – TUT 5x3" would result in a 5 second lowering phase, followed by 3 seconds lifting to return to starting position.

For TUT movements aim to complete at the very least 2 repetitions but ideally 4.

After completing the full circuit rest 60 seconds before repeating.

Wait 90 seconds between moving from one circuit to the next.

Circuit 1: x3

Air Squats	TUT 5x3
Pike Push-ups	TUT 5x3
Reverse Lunges	TUT 5x3
Single Leg Glute	TUT 5x3
Plank	45 secs

Circuit 2: x3

Jumping Lunges	8 reps
Hindu Push-ups	8-10 reps
Calf Raises & Hold	12 reps
Shoulder Rotations	45 secs
Side Plank	35 secs
Reverse Lunges	8 reps

Circuit 3: x2

Diamond Push-ups	5-7 reps
Ab Hold	8 reps
Air Squats	8-10 reps

Circuit 1: x3

Under Table Row	TUT 5x3
Reverse Lunges	10 reps
Leg Raises & Hold	8 reps
Towel Bicep Curl	TUT 5x3
Single Leg Glute	8 reps

Circuit 2: x3

Under Table Row	TUT 5x3
Side Plank	35 secs
Push-ups	8-10 reps
Back Extension	6 reps
Towel Twist	12-15 reps
Shoulder Rotations	45 secs

Circuit 3: x2

Pike Push-ups	12 reps
Towel Bicep Curl	12 reps
Air Squats	8 reps

Session 3

Circuit 1: x3

Push-ups	TUT 5x3
Plank	45 secs
Jump Squats	8 reps
Tricep Wall Press	TUT 5x3
Reverse Lunges	6-8 reps

Circuit 2: x3

Lunges	7-10 reps
Pike Push-ups	TUT 5x3
Diamond Push-ups	5 reps
Leg Raises	10 reps

Circuit 3: x3

Incline Push-ups	8-10 reps
Superman	5 reps
Glute Bridge & Hold	10 reps

Circuit 1: x3
No rest between exercises

Mountain Climbers	30 reps
Leg Raises	12 reps
Mountain Climbers	20 reps
Crunches	10 reps
Mountain Climbers	15 reps
Side Jack Knife	7 reps

Complete each exercise in the order listed below.

Aim for the target repetitions (reps) specified and depending on fitness level rest 30-45 seconds between exercises. Repeat the circuit for the specified number, i.e. "*Circuit 1: x4*" means that you will repeat this circuit 4 times before moving onto the next circuit.

Where you see "LAT", this tells you that it is a Lactic Acid Training style exercise.

"Air Squats – LAT 5 reps" would result in a 1 second lowering phase, followed by 3-4 seconds lifting to return to starting position, repeated 5 times.

For LAT movements aim to perform the lowering phase as fast as possible whilst still being under control and in good form.

After completing the full circuit rest 60 seconds before repeating.

Wait 90 seconds between moving from one circuit to the next.

Circuit 1: x3

Air Squats	LAT 6-8 reps
Push-ups	LAT 6-8 reps
Star Jumps	15 reps
Reverse Lunges	LAT 8 reps
Calf Raises	LAT 10-12 reps

Circuit 2: x3

Burpees	8 reps
Crunches	15 reps
Jumping Lunges	8-10 reps
Side-to-Side Push-ups	10 reps
Side Plank	45 secs

Circuit 3: x2

Pike Push-ups	LAT 6-8 reps
Reverse Lunges	5 reps
High Knees	12-15 reps
Single Leg Glute	LAT 8 reps
Arms Extended Crunch	10 reps

Circuit 1: x3

Wide Grip Table Row	LAT 5 reps
Leg Raises & Hold	6 reps
Bicep Towel Curl	LAT 6 reps
Jump Squats	10 reps
Hindu Push-ups	6-8 reps
Superman	6 reps

Circuit 2: x3

Close Grip Table Row	LAT 5 reps
Skipping	30 secs
Push-ups with Twist	8 reps
Advanced Tricep Press	6 reps

Circuit 3: x2

Reverse Lunges	10 reps
Mountain Climbers	15 reps
Bicep Towel Curl	LAT 4-6 reps
Towel Twist	10 reps
Bicep Towel Curl	10 reps

Circuit 1: x3

Push-ups	LAT 6-8 reps
Plank	45 secs
Diamond Push-ups	LAT 5 reps
Toe Touchers	8-10 reps
Single Leg Glute	12 reps

Circuit 2: x3

Hindu Push-ups	12-15 reps
Air Squats	10 reps
Incline Push-ups	LAT 6 reps
Calf Raises	20 reps
Explosive Tricep Press	5 reps

Circuit 3: x2

Spiderman Push-ups	8 reps
Mountain Climbers	20 reps
Back Extension	6 reps
Side-to-Side Push-ups	8 reps

Session 4

Circuit 1: x2

Star Jumps	10 reps
Skipping	45 secs
Mountain Climbers	20 reps

Circuit 2: x1

Burpees	10 reps

Circuit 3: x1

Plank	30 secs
Arms Extended Crunch	10 reps
Toe Touchers	10 reps

Circuit 4: x1

Side Plank	30 secs
Jack Knife	10 reps
Ab Hold	5 reps

Complete each exercise in the order listed below.

Aim for the target repetitions (reps) specified and depending on fitness level rest 20-30 seconds between exercises. Repeat the circuit for the specified number, i.e. *"Circuit 1: x4"* means that you will repeat this circuit 4 times before moving onto the next circuit.

Where you see "LAT", this tells you that it is a Lactic Acid Training style exercise.

"Air Squats – LAT 5 reps" would result in a 1 second lowering phase, followed by 3-4 seconds lifting to return to starting position, repeated 5 times.

For LAT movements aim to perform the lowering phase as fast as possible whilst still being under control and in good form.

After completing the full circuit rest 30-45 seconds before repeating.

Wait 45-60 seconds between moving from one circuit to the next.

Circuit 1: x3

Air Squats	LAT 8 reps
Side to Side Push-ups	LAT 8 reps
Mountain Climbers	25 reps
Reverse Lunges	LAT 8 reps

Circuit 2: x3

Burpees	12 reps
Jumping Lunges	8-10 reps
Hindu Push-ups	10 reps
Plank	60 secs

Circuit 3: x2

Pike Push-ups	LAT 6 reps
Air Squats	15 reps
Mountain Climbers	25 reps
Single Leg Glute	LAT 6 reps
Crunches	10 reps

Circuit 1: x3

Wide Grip Table Row	LAT 6 reps
Leg Raises & Hold	8 reps
Bicep Towel Curl	LAT 6 reps
Air Squats	10 reps
Pike Push-ups	8 reps
Ab Hold	8 reps

Circuit 2: x3

Close Grip Table Row	LAT 5 reps
Star Jumps	15 reps
Push-ups with Twist	8 reps
Tricep Press	10 reps

Circuit 3: x2

Reverse Lunges	10 reps
Bicep Towel Curl	LAT 4-6 reps
Towel Twist	10 reps

Circuit 1: x3

Push-ups	LAT 6-8 reps
Plank	45 secs
Tricep Wall Press	LAT 5 reps
Toe Touchers	8-10 reps
Single Leg Glute	12 reps

Circuit 2: x3

Pike Push-ups	LAT 6 reps
Crunches	10 reps
Side to Side Push-ups	LAT 6 reps
Mountain Climbers	20 reps
Diamond Push-ups	8 reps

Circuit 3: x2

Reverse Lunges	10 reps
Star Jumps	10 reps
Ab Hold	8 reps
Side-to-Side Push-ups	6 reps

Session 4

Circuit 1: x2

Star Jumps	15 reps
Skipping	30 secs
Mountain Climbers	25 reps

Circuit 2: x1

Burpees	10 reps

Circuit 3: x1

Plank	45 secs
Arms Extended Crunch	12 reps
Toe Touchers	10 reps

Circuit 4: x1

Side Plank	45 secs
Jack Knife	10 reps
Ab Hold	5 reps
Arms Extended Crunch	8 reps

Complete each exercise in the order listed below.

Aim for the target repetitions (reps) specified and depending on fitness level rest 30-45 seconds between exercises. Repeat the circuit for the specified number, i.e. "*Circuit 1: x4*" means that you will repeat this circuit 4 times before moving onto the next circuit.

Where you see "TUT", this stands for time under tension and states the length of time for a given exercise. So, TUT 5x3 would mean 5 seconds for the first part of the exercise followed by 3 seconds for the second part i.e.:

"Air Squats – TUT 5x3" would result in a 5 second lowering phase, followed by 3 seconds lifting to return to starting position.

For TUT movements aim to complete at the very least 2 repetitions but ideally 4.

After completing the full circuit rest 50 seconds before repeating.

Wait 70 seconds between moving from one circuit to the next.

Circuit 1: x3

Air Squats	TUT 5x4
Pike Push-ups	TUT 5x4
Reverse Lunges	TUT 5x3
Single Leg Glute	TUT 5x3
Plank	45 secs

Circuit 2: x3

Jumping Lunges	8 reps
Hindu Push-ups	8-10 reps
Calf Raises & Hold	12 reps
Shoulder Rotations	45 secs
Side Plank	35 secs
Reverse Lunges	8 reps

Circuit 3: x2

Diamond Push-ups	5-7 reps
Ab Hold	8 reps
Air Squats	8-10 reps

Circuit 1: x3

Under Table Row	TUT 5x4
Reverse Lunges	10 reps
Leg Raises & Hold	8 reps
Towel Bicep Curl	TUT 5x4
Single Leg Glute	8 reps

Circuit 2: x3

Under Table Row	TUT 5x3
Side Plank	35 secs
Push-ups	8-10 reps
Back Extension	6 reps
Towel Twist	12-15 reps
Shoulder Rotations	45 secs

Circuit 3: x2

Pike Push-ups	12 reps
Towel Bicep Curl	12 reps
Air Squats	8 reps

Session 3

Circuit 1: x3

Push-ups	TUT 5x4
Plank	45 secs
Jump Squats	8 reps
Tricep Wall Press	TUT 5x4
Reverse Lunges	6-8 reps

Circuit 2: x3

Lunges	7-10 reps
Pike Push-ups	TUT 5x4
Diamond Push-ups	5 reps
Leg Raises	10 reps

Circuit 3: x3

Incline Push-ups	8-10 reps
Superman	5 reps
Glute Bridge & Hold	10 reps

Circuit 1: x3
No rest between exercises

Mountain Climbers	30 reps
Leg Raises	12 reps
Mountain Climbers	20 reps
Crunches	10 reps
Mountain Climbers	15 reps
Side Jack Knife	7 reps

Complete each exercise in the order listed below.

Aim for the target repetitions (reps) specified and depending on fitness level rest 20-30 seconds between exercises. Repeat the circuit for the specified number, i.e. *"Circuit 1: x4"* means that you will repeat this circuit 4 times before moving onto the next circuit.

Where you see "LAT", this tells you that it is a Lactic Acid Training style exercise.

"Air Squats – LAT 5 reps" would result in a 1 second lowering phase, followed by 3-4 seconds lifting to return to starting position, repeated 5 times.

For LAT movements aim to perform the lowering phase as fast as possible whilst still being under control and in good form.

After completing the full circuit rest 30 seconds before repeating.

Wait 45 seconds between moving from one circuit to the next.

Circuit 1: x3

Air Squats	LAT 8 reps
Side to Side Push-ups	LAT 8 reps
Mountain Climbers	25 reps
Reverse Lunges	LAT 8 reps

Circuit 2: x3

Burpees	12 reps
Jumping Lunges	8-10 reps
Hindu Push-ups	10 reps
Plank	60 secs

Circuit 3: x2

Pike Push-ups	LAT 6 reps
Air Squats	15 reps
Mountain Climbers	25 reps
Single Leg Glute	LAT 6 reps
Crunches	10 reps

Circuit 1: x3

Wide Grip Table Row	LAT 6 reps
Leg Raises & Hold	8 reps
Bicep Towel Curl	LAT 6 reps
Air Squats	10 reps
Pike Push-ups	8 reps
Ab Hold	8 reps

Circuit 2: x3

Close Grip Table Row	LAT 5 reps
Star Jumps	15 reps
Push-ups with Twist	8 reps
Tricep Press	10 reps

Circuit 3: x2

Reverse Lunges	10 reps
Bicep Towel Curl	LAT 4-6 reps
Towel Twist	10 reps

Circuit 1: x3

Push-ups	LAT 6-8 reps
Plank	45 secs
Tricep Wall Press	LAT 5 reps
Toe Touchers	8-10 reps
Single Leg Glute	12 reps

Circuit 2: x3

Pike Push-ups	LAT 6 reps
Crunches	10 reps
Side to Side Push-ups	LAT 6 reps
Mountain Climbers	20 reps
Diamond Push-ups	8 reps

Circuit 3: x2

Reverse Lunges	10 reps
Star Jumps	10 reps
Ab Hold	8 reps
Side-to-Side Push-ups	6 reps

Session 4

Circuit 1: x2

Star Jumps	15 reps
Skipping	30 secs
Mountain Climbers	25 reps

Circuit 2: x1

Burpees	10 reps

Circuit 3: x1

Plank	45 secs
Arms Extended Crunch	12 reps
Toe Touchers	10 reps

Circuit 4: x1

Side Plank	45 secs
Jack Knife	10 reps
Ab Hold	5 reps
Arms Extended Crunch	8 reps

Complete each exercise in the order listed below.

Aim for the target repetitions (reps) specified and depending on fitness level rest 0-30 seconds between exercises.
Repeat the circuit for the specified number, i.e. "*Circuit 1: x4*" means that you will repeat this circuit 4 times before moving onto the next circuit.

After completing the full circuit rest 30-60 seconds before repeating.

Wait 60-90 seconds between moving from one circuit to the next.

Session 1

Circuit 1: x4

Air Squats	20-25 reps
Pike Push-ups	12-15 reps
Plank	35-45 secs
Glute Bridge & Hold	15 reps
Lunges	10-12 reps

Circuit 2: x3

Push-ups	15-20 reps
Reverse Lunges	12-15 reps
Calf Raises & Hold	15 reps
Shoulder Rotations	60 secs
Side Plank	30 secs
Air Squats	15-20 reps

Circuit 3: x3

Pike Push-ups	12-15 reps
Shoulder Rotation	45 secs
Diamond Push-ups	12-15 reps
Jump Squats	8 reps

Circuit 1: x4

Reverse Lunges	15 reps
Leg Raises	10-12 reps
Wide Grip Table Row	8-10 reps
Towel Bicep Curl	15 reps
Single Leg Glute	10 reps

Circuit 2: x4

Close Grip Table Row	8-10 reps
Plank	30 secs
Wide Push-ups	12-15 reps
Superman	8 reps
Towel Twist	15 reps

Circuit 3: x3

Jump Squats	5 reps
Pike Push-ups	10-12 reps
Towel Bicep Curl	15 reps
Superman	8 reps

Session 3

Circuit 1: x4

Air Squats	10 reps
Push-ups	15-20 reps
Plank	30 secs
Diamond Push-ups	10-12 reps
Towel Bicep Curl	8-10 reps

Circuit 2: x3

Reverse Lunges	10 reps
Incline Push-ups	10-12 reps
Tricep Wall Press	10-15 reps
Leg Raises	10 reps

Circuit 3: x3

Wide Push-ups	8-10 reps
Superman	8 reps

Circuit 1: x3

High Knees	25 reps
Mountain Climbers	35 reps
Leg Raises	10-15 reps
Crunches	25 reps
Plank	60 secs
Skipping	90 secs

Complete each exercise in the order listed below.

Aim for the target repetitions (reps) specified and depending on fitness level rest 0-30 seconds between exercises.
Repeat the circuit for the specified number, i.e. *"Circuit 1: x4"* means that you will repeat this circuit 4 times before moving onto the next circuit.

After completing the full circuit rest 30 seconds before repeating.

Wait 60 seconds between moving from one circuit to the next.

Circuit 1: x4

Air Squats	25-30 reps
Pike Push-ups	15-20 reps
Plank	45 secs
Glute Bridge & Hold	15 reps
Lunges	12-15 reps

Circuit 2: x3

Push-ups	20 reps
Reverse Lunges	15 reps
Calf Raises & Hold	20 reps
Shoulder Rotations	60 secs
Side Plank	30 secs
Air Squats	20 reps

Circuit 3: x3

Pike Push-ups	15-20 reps
Shoulder Rotation	45 secs
Diamond Push-ups	15 reps
Jump Squats	8 reps

Circuit 1: x4

Reverse Lunges	15-20 reps
Leg Raises & Hold	8 reps
Wide Grip Table Row	10 reps
Towel Bicep Curl	15 reps
Single Leg Glute	10 reps

Circuit 2: x4

Close Grip Table Row	10 reps
Side Plank	30 secs
Wide Push-ups	15 reps
Superman	8 reps
Towel Twist	15 reps

Circuit 3: x3

Jump Squats	8 reps
Pike Push-ups	12-15 reps
Towel Bicep Curl	15 reps
Superman	8 reps

Session 3

Circuit 1: x4

Air Squats	15 reps
Push-ups	20 reps
Plank	45 secs
Diamond Push-ups	12 reps
Towel Bicep Curl	10 reps

Circuit 2: x3

Reverse Lunges	12-15 reps
Incline Push-ups	15-20 reps
Tricep Wall Press	20-25 reps
Leg Raises & Hold	5-8 reps

Circuit 3: x3

Wide Push-ups	10-12 reps
Superman	8 reps

Session 4

Circuit 1: x3

High Knees	25 reps
Mountain Climbers	35 reps
Leg Raises	10-15 reps
Crunches	25 reps
Plank	60 secs
Skipping	90 secs

Circuit 2

Burpees	Until failure

Complete each exercise in the order listed below.

Aim for the target repetitions (reps) specified and depending on fitness level rest 30-45 seconds between exercises. Repeat the circuit for the specified number, i.e. "*Circuit 1: x4*" means that you will repeat this circuit 4 times before moving onto the next circuit.

Where you see "TUT", this stands for time under tension and states the length of time for a given exercise. So, TUT 5x3 would mean 5 seconds for the first part of the exercise followed by 3 seconds for the second part i.e.:

"Air Squats – TUT 5x3" would result in a 5 second lowering phase, followed by 3 seconds lifting to return to starting position.

For TUT movements aim to complete at the very least 4 repetitions but ideally 6.

After completing the full circuit rest 60-90 seconds before repeating.

Wait 90 seconds between moving from one circuit to the next.

Circuit 1: x3

Air Squats	TUT 3x3
Pike Push-ups	TUT 3x3
Reverse Lunges	TUT 3x3
Single Leg Glute	TUT 3x3
Plank	45 secs

Circuit 2: x3

Jumping Lunges	10 reps
Hindu Push-ups	12-15 reps
Calf Raises & Hold	15 reps
Shoulder Rotations	60 secs
Side Plank	45 secs
Reverse Lunges	10-15 reps

Circuit 3: x3

Diamond Push-ups	10-12 reps
Ab Hold	10 reps
Jump Squats	5 reps

Circuit 1: x4

Wide Grip Table Row	TUT 3x3
Reverse Lunges	10-12 reps
Leg Raises & Hold	8-10 reps
Towel Bicep Curl	TUT 3x3
Single Leg Glute	8 reps

Circuit 2: x3

Close Grip Table Row	TUT 3x3
Side Plank	35 secs
Wide Push-ups	15 reps
Back Extension	5 reps
Towel Twist	12 reps
Shoulder Rotations	60 secs

Circuit 3: x2

Hindu Push-ups	15 reps
Towel Bicep Curl	15 reps
Air Squats	10-12 reps

Session 3

Circuit 1: x4

Push-ups	TUT 3x3
Plank	30 secs
Jump Squats	8-10 reps
Diamond Push-ups	TUT 3x3
Reverse Lunges	5 reps

Circuit 2: x3

Lunges	10 reps
Pike Push-ups	TUT 3x3
Diamond Push-ups	5 reps
Leg raises	10 reps
Side Plank	30 secs

Circuit 3: x3

Incline Push-ups	10 reps
Superman	8 reps
Glute Bridge & Hold	10-12 reps

Circuit 1: x3
No rest between exercises

Mountain Climbers	30 reps
Leg Raises	15 reps
Mountain Climbers	30 reps
Crunches	12 reps
Mountain Climbers	30 reps
Side Jack Knife	10 reps

Complete each exercise in the order listed below.

Aim for the target repetitions (reps) specified and depending on fitness level rest 30-45 seconds between exercises. Repeat the circuit for the specified number, i.e. *"Circuit 1: x4"* means that you will repeat this circuit 4 times before moving onto the next circuit.

Where you see "TUT", this stands for time under tension and states the length of time for a given exercise. So, TUT 5x3 would mean 5 seconds for the first part of the exercise followed by 3 seconds for the second part i.e.:

"Air Squats – TUT 5x3" would result in a 5 second lowering phase, followed by 3 seconds lifting to return to starting position.

For TUT movements aim to complete at the very least 4 repetitions but ideally 6.

After completing the full circuit rest 60-90 seconds before repeating.

Wait 90 seconds between moving from one circuit to the next.

Circuit 1: x3

Air Squats	TUT 4x4
Pike Push-ups	TUT 4x4
Reverse Lunges	TUT 4x4
Single Leg Glute	TUT 4x4
Plank	60 secs

Circuit 2: x3

Jumping Lunges	12 reps
Hindu Push-ups	15-18 reps
Calf Raises & Hold	20 reps
Shoulder Rotations	60 secs
Side Plank	60 secs
Reverse Lunges	15 reps

Circuit 3: x3

Diamond Push-ups	12-15 reps
Ab Hold	12 reps
Jump Squats	8 reps

Circuit 1: x4

Wide Grip Table Row	TUT 4x4
Reverse Lunges	12-15 reps
Leg Raises & Hold	10 reps
Towel Bicep Curl	TUT 4x4
Single Leg Glute	12 reps

Circuit 2: x3

Close Grip Table Row	TUT 4x4
Side Plank	45 secs
Wide Push-ups	20-25 reps
Back Extension	8 reps
Towel Twist	15 reps
Shoulder Rotations	60 secs

Circuit 3: x2

Hindu Push-ups	20 reps
Towel Bicep Curl	15 reps
Air Squats	12 reps

Session 3

Circuit 1: x4

Push-ups	TUT 4x4
Plank	45 secs
Jump Squats	10 reps
Diamond Push-ups	TUT 4x4
Reverse Lunges	10 reps

Circuit 2: x3

Lunges	10 reps
Pike Push-ups	TUT 4x4
Diamond Push-ups	8 reps
Leg raises	12 reps
Side Plank	45 secs

Circuit 3: x3

Incline Push-ups	15-20 reps
Superman	8 reps
Glute Bridge & Hold	12 reps

Circuit 1: x3
No rest between exercises

Mountain Climbers	30 reps
Leg Raises	15 reps
Mountain Climbers	30 reps
Crunches	12 reps
Mountain Climbers	30 reps
Side Jack Knife	10 reps

Circuit 2: x2

Burpees	Until failure

Complete each exercise in the order listed below.

Aim for the target repetitions (reps) specified and depending on fitness level rest 30-45 seconds between exercises. Repeat the circuit for the specified number, i.e. *"Circuit 1: x4"* means that you will repeat this circuit 4 times before moving onto the next circuit.

Where you see "LAT", this tells you that it is a Lactic Acid Training style exercise.

"Air Squats – LAT 5 reps" would result in a 1 second lowering phase, followed by 3-4 seconds lifting to return to starting position, repeated 5 times.

For LAT movements aim to perform the lowering phase as fast as possible whilst still being under control and in good form.

After completing the full circuit rest 60 seconds before repeating.

Wait 90 seconds between moving from one circuit to the next.

Circuit 1: x4

Air Squats	LAT 8-10 reps
Push-ups	LAT 8-10 reps
Star Jumps	25-30 reps
Reverse Lunges	LAT 10 reps
Calf Raises	LAT 15 reps

Circuit 2: x3

Burpees	12 reps
Crunches	20-25 reps
Jumping Lunges	12 reps
Side-to-Side Push-ups	12-16 reps
Side Plank	60 secs

Circuit 3: x2

Wall Shoulder Push-ups	10 reps
Reverse Lunges	12 reps
High Knees	20 reps
Single Leg Glute	LAT 12-15 reps
Arms Extended Crunch	20 reps

Circuit 1: x4

Wide Grip Table Row	LAT 8-10 reps
Leg Raises & Hold	12-15 reps
Bicep Towel Curl	LAT 10 reps
Jump Squats	15 reps
Wall Shoulder Push-ups	8-12 reps
Superman	8 reps

Circuit 2: x3

Close Grip Table Row	LAT 8-10 reps
Skipping	60 secs
Push-ups with Twist	10-12 reps
Advanced Tricep Press	8-10 reps

Circuit 3: x2

Reverse Lunges	12 reps
Mountain Climbers	20 reps
Bicep Towel Curl	LAT 6-8 reps
Towel Twist	15 reps
Bicep Towel Curl	15 reps

Session 3

Circuit 1: x3

Push-ups	LAT 10-12 reps
Plank	60 secs
Diamond Push-ups	LAT 8 reps
Toe Touchers	12 reps
Single Leg Glute	15 reps

Circuit 2: x3

Hindu Push-ups	15-20 reps
Jump Squats	6 reps
Incline Push-ups	LAT 8 reps
Calf Raises	20 reps
Explosive Tricep Press	10 reps

Circuit 3: x2

Spiderman Push-ups	12 reps
Mountain Climbers	20 reps
Back Extension	6 reps
Side-to-Side Push-ups	12 reps

Session 4

Circuit 1: x2

Star Jumps	20 reps
Skipping	90 secs
Mountain Climbers	20 reps

Circuit 2: x1

Burpees	12 reps

Circuit 3: x1

Plank	60 secs
Arms Extended Crunch	15 reps
Toe Touchers	15 reps

Circuit 4: x1

Side Plank	60 secs
Jack Knife	15 reps
Ab Hold	12 reps

Complete each exercise in the order listed below.

Aim for the target repetitions (reps) specified and depending on fitness level rest 30 seconds between exercises. Repeat the circuit for the specified number, i.e. *"Circuit 1: x4"* means that you will repeat this circuit 4 times before moving onto the next circuit.

Where you see "LAT", this tells you that it is a Lactic Acid Training style exercise.

"Air Squats – LAT 5 reps" would result in a 1 second lowering phase, followed by 3-4 seconds lifting to return to starting position, repeated 5 times.

For LAT movements aim to perform the lowering phase as fast as possible whilst still being under control and in good form.

After completing the full circuit rest 60 seconds before repeating.

Wait 45-60 seconds between moving from one circuit to the next.

Circuit 1: x4

Air Squats	LAT 8 reps
Side to Side Push-ups	LAT 8 reps
Mountain Climbers	35 reps
Reverse Lunges	LAT 8 reps

Circuit 2: x4

Burpees	15 reps
Jumping Lunges	10 reps
Hindu Push-ups	12 reps
Plank	70 secs

Circuit 3: x2

Pike Push-ups	LAT 8 reps
Air Squats	20 reps
Mountain Climbers	20 reps
Single Leg Glute	LAT 8 reps
Crunches	20 reps

Session 2

Circuit 1: x4

Wide Grip Table Row	LAT 6 reps
Leg Raises & Hold	15 reps
Bicep Towel Curl	LAT 8 reps
Air Squats	15 reps
Pike Push-ups	12 reps
Ab Hold	10 reps

Circuit 2: x3

Close Grip Table Row	LAT 8 reps
Star Jumps	10 reps
Push-ups with Twist	15 reps
Tricep Wall Press	10 reps

Circuit 3: x2

Reverse Lunges	12 reps
Bicep Towel Curl	LAT 6-8 reps
Crunches	15 reps
Towel Twist	10 reps

Session 3

Circuit 1: x4

Push-ups	LAT 8 reps
Plank	60 secs
Tricep Wall Press	LAT 6 reps
Toe Touchers	10 reps
Single Leg Glute	15 reps

Circuit 2: x3

Pike Push-ups	LAT 6 reps
Arms Extended Crunch	10 reps
Side to Side Push-ups	12 reps
Mountain Climbers	25 reps
Diamond Push-ups	12 reps

Circuit 3: x2

Reverse Lunges	12 reps
Star Jumps	15 reps
Ab Hold	10 reps
Side-to-Side Push-ups	6 reps
Plank	60 secs

Session 4

Circuit 1: x2

Star Jumps	25 reps
Skipping	60 secs
Mountain Climbers	35 reps

Circuit 2: x1

Burpees	15 reps

Circuit 3: x1

Plank	60 secs
Arms Extended Crunch	15 reps
Toe Touchers	12 reps

Circuit 4: x1

Side Plank	45 secs
Jack Knife	10 reps
Ab Hold	5 reps
Arms Extended Crunch	8 reps

Complete each exercise in the order listed below.

Aim for the target repetitions (reps) specified and depending on fitness level rest 30-45 seconds between exercises. Repeat the circuit for the specified number, i.e. *"Circuit 1: x4"* means that you will repeat this circuit 4 times before moving onto the next circuit.

Where you see "TUT", this stands for time under tension and states the length of time for a given exercise. So, TUT 5x3 would mean 5 seconds for the first part of the exercise followed by 3 seconds for the second part i.e.:

"Air Squats – TUT 5x3" would result in a 5 second lowering phase, followed by 3 seconds lifting to return to starting position.

For TUT movements aim to complete at the very least 4 repetitions but ideally 6.

After completing the full circuit rest 60-80 seconds before repeating.

Wait 90 seconds between moving from one circuit to the next.

Session 1

Circuit 1: x3

Air Squats	TUT 5x5
Pike Push-ups	TUT 5x5
Reverse Lunges	TUT 5x5
Single Leg Glute	TUT 5x5
Plank	70 secs

Circuit 2: x3

Jumping Lunges	15 reps
Hindu Push-ups	15 reps
Calf Raises & Hold	15 reps
Shoulder Rotations	60 secs
Side Plank	45 secs
Reverse Lunges	15 reps

Circuit 3: x3

Diamond Push-ups	15 reps
Ab Hold	12 reps
Jump Squats	10 reps

Session 2

Circuit 1: x4

Wide Grip Table Row	TUT 5x5
Reverse Lunges	12-15 reps
Leg Raises & Hold	10 reps
Towel Bicep Curl	TUT 4x4
Single Leg Glute	12 reps

Circuit 2: x3

Close Grip Table Row	TUT 4x4
Side Plank	45 secs
Wide Push-ups	20-25 reps
Back Extension	8 reps
Towel Twist	15 reps
Shoulder Rotations	60 secs

Circuit 3: x2

Hindu Push-ups	20 reps
Towel Bicep Curl	15 reps
Air Squats	12 reps

Circuit 1: x4

Push-ups	TUT 5x5
Plank	45 secs
Jump Squats	10 reps
Diamond Push-ups	TUT 5x5
Reverse Lunges	10 reps

Circuit 2: x3

Lunges	10 reps
Pike Push-ups	TUT 5x5
Diamond Push-ups	8 reps
Leg raises	12 reps
Side Plank	45 secs

Circuit 3: x3

Incline Push-ups	15-20 reps
Superman	8 reps
Glute Bridge & Hold	12 reps

Circuit 1: x3
No rest between exercises

Mountain Climbers	30 reps
Leg Raises	15 reps
Mountain Climbers	30 reps
Crunches	12 reps
Mountain Climbers	30 reps
Side Jack Knife	10 reps

Circuit 2: x2

Burpees	Until failure

Complete each exercise in the order listed below.

Aim for the target repetitions (reps) specified and depending on fitness level rest 30 seconds between exercises. Repeat the circuit for the specified number, i.e. *"Circuit 1: x4"* means that you will repeat this circuit 4 times before moving onto the next circuit.

Where you see "LAT", this tells you that it is a Lactic Acid Training style exercise.

"Air Squats – LAT 5 reps" would result in a 1 second lowering phase, followed by 3-4 seconds lifting to return to starting position, repeated 5 times.

For LAT movements aim to perform the lowering phase as fast as possible whilst still being under control and in good form.

After completing the full circuit rest 45 seconds before repeating.

Wait 45 seconds between moving from one circuit to the next.

Circuit 1: x4

Air Squats	LAT 8 reps
Side to Side Push-ups	LAT 8 reps
Mountain Climbers	35 reps
Reverse Lunges	LAT 8 reps

Circuit 2: x4

Burpees	15 reps
Jumping Lunges	10 reps
Hindu Push-ups	12 reps
Plank	70 secs

Circuit 3: x2

Pike Push-ups	LAT 8 reps
Air Squats	20 reps
Mountain Climbers	20 reps
Single Leg Glute	LAT 8 reps
Crunches	20 reps

Circuit 1: x4

Wide Grip Table Row	LAT 6 reps
Leg Raises & Hold	15 reps
Bicep Towel Curl	LAT 8 reps
Air Squats	15 reps
Pike Push-ups	12 reps
Ab Hold	10 reps

Circuit 2: x3

Close Grip Table Row	LAT 8 reps
Star Jumps	10 reps
Push-ups with Twist	15 reps
Tricep Wall Press	10 reps

Circuit 3: x2

Reverse Lunges	12 reps
Bicep Towel Curl	LAT 6-8 reps
Crunches	15 reps
Towel Twist	10 reps

Circuit 1: x4

Push-ups	LAT 8 reps
Plank	60 secs
Tricep Wall Press	LAT 6 reps
Toe Touchers	10 reps
Single Leg Glute	15 reps

Circuit 2: x3

Pike Push-ups	LAT 6 reps
Arms Extended Crunch	10 reps
Side to Side Push-ups	12 reps
Mountain Climbers	25 reps
Diamond Push-ups	12 reps

Circuit 3: x2

Reverse Lunges	12 reps
Star Jumps	15 reps
Ab Hold	10 reps
Side-to-Side Push-ups	6 reps
Plank	60 secs

Session 4

Circuit 1: x2

Star Jumps	25 reps
Skipping	60 secs
Mountain Climbers	35 reps

Circuit 2: x1

Burpees	15 reps

Circuit 3: x1

Plank	60 secs
Arms Extended Crunch	15 reps
Toe Touchers	12 reps

Circuit 4: x1

Side Plank	45 secs
Jack Knife	10 reps
Ab Hold	5 reps
Arms Extended Crunch	8 reps

Your Free Gift

I wanted to show my appreciation that you support my work so I've put together a free gift for you.

The 'Your Body is Your Gym' Bonus Pack

Just visit the link below to download it now.

www.GoodLivingPublishing.com/bodyweight

I know you will love this gift.

Thanks!

Peter Paulson

Made in the USA
Middletown, DE
08 April 2021